Rubber Dam
Medium Green Latex Squares

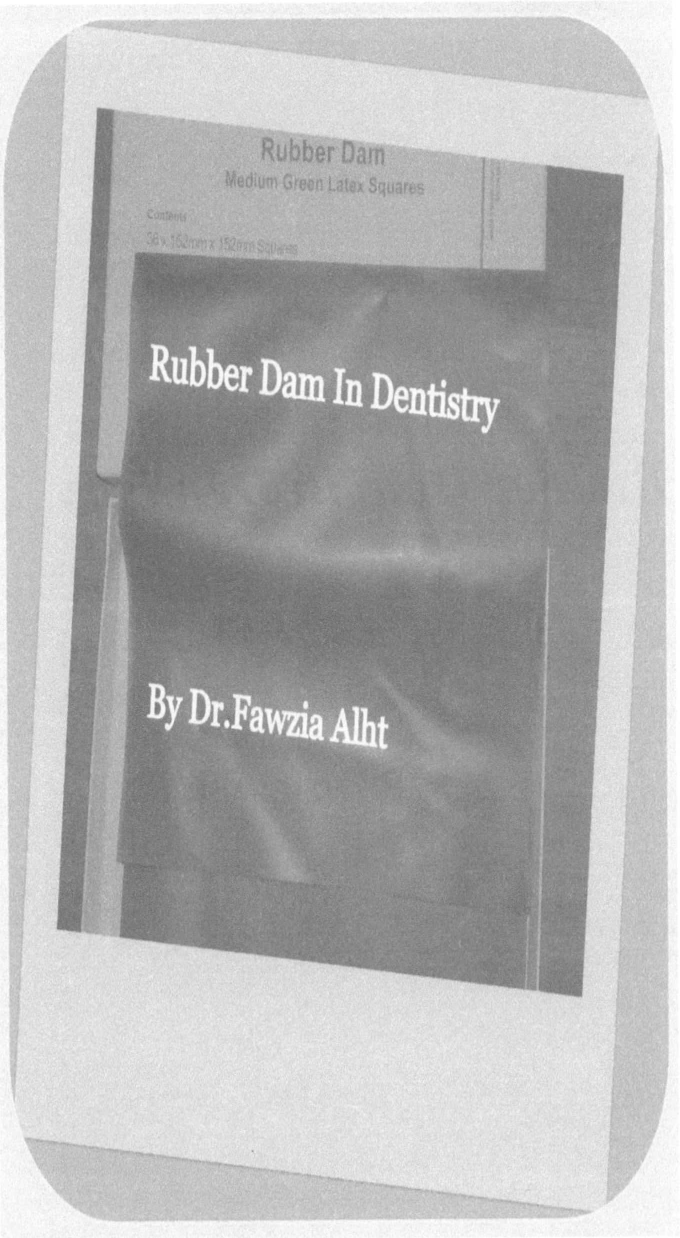

Contents
36 x 152mm x 152mm Squares

Rubber Dam In Dentistry

By Dr.Fawzia Alht

Rubber Dam in Dentistry

By Dr. Fawzia Alht

Table of The contents

Introduction

This book gives you the practical and the essential
information of Rubber Dam in Dentistry. It
is written in a simple language with ample
photos support. This book provides guidance
in step wise manner .It is a ready reference
guide for the young students and general
students. This book is written by a female
Yemeni general dentist .

Rubber Dam Isolation

In 1864 ,S.C Barnum a dentist in New York introduced a rubber dam into dentistry .Use of the rubber dam ensures appropriate dryness of the teeth and improves the quality of
clinical restorative dentistry .The rubber dam is used to eliminate saliva and retract soft tissue.

Advantages of The Rubber dam

- Patient protection and reduce risk: Using rubber dam prevent patient to swallow the debris and foreign objects ,so the restorative procedures is more comfortable and relaxed.

- Increase Access and visibility : Using rubber dam remove the visual obstruction during restorative procedures(the cheeks, lips , and tongue).And operative visibility is greatly improved.

- Improved Time efficiency: Using Rubber dam provides clear restorative field with greater efficiency .

- Moisture control and improved the quality of dental materials that are affected by saliva. However, rubber dam using enhances a moisture-free , uncontaminated working free environment. The quality of result of the restoration is highly superior to those that are performed without dental dam utilization .

Rubber Dam Materials

Rubber dam are available in latex and non latex .

Also , dark and light dam materials .The darker one gives better contrast .The Rubber dam has a shiny side and dull one. The dull one is light reflective and it is placed facing the occlusal side of the isolated teeth .The thicker dam is more effective in retracting the tissue and more resistant to tearing especially in class v lesion with cervical retainer .While the thinner material has the advantage of passing through the contacts easier particularly when the contacts are tight.

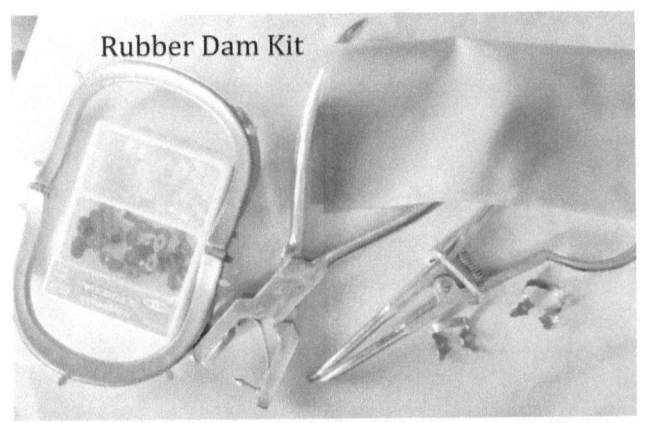

Rubber Dam Kit

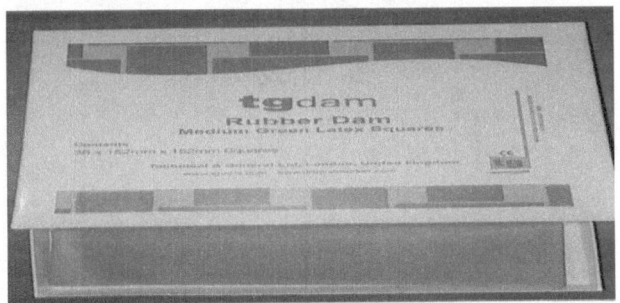

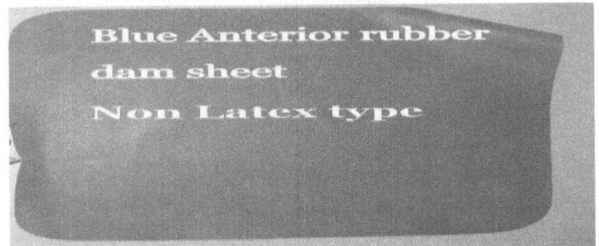

Blue Anterior rubber dam sheet

Non Latex type

Clamps:

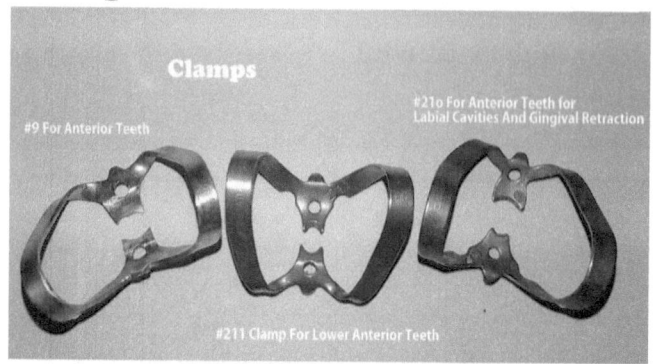

Clamps

#9 For Anterior Teeth

#21o For Anterior Teeth for Labial Cavities And Gingival Retraction

#211 Clamp For Lower Anterior Teeth

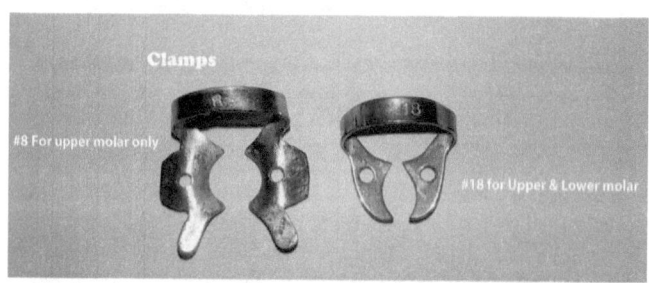

Clamps

#8 For upper molar only

#18 for Upper & Lower molar

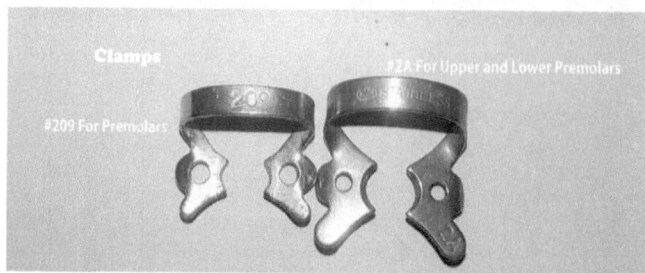

Clamps

#209 For Premolars

#2A For Upper and Lower Premolars

There are variety of clamps . The above photos show the clamps I choose to use always. There are wingless clamps or retainer and clamps without wings. The wings provide extra retraction for the rubber dam .No.9 clamp or retainer for anterior teeth is applied after the rubber dam is in place or you can place it first ,then stretch the dam over it (that is my favorite method in placing it) .For extra security , dental floss is utilized if the clamps are accidentally

swallowed or aspirated. Also,in general sometimes it is necessary to grind recontour the jaws of the retainer to the shape of the tooth by grinding with a mounted stone. Moreover, there are plastic clamps which are used when metal clamps obstruction is a problem in radiography because radiolucent plastic clamps allow for an unobstructed view of the tooth .Additionally, plastic clamps are used to isolate the teeth during vital tooth bleaching.

Clamp Selection

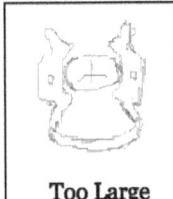 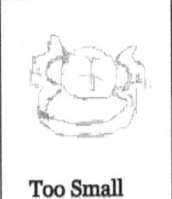 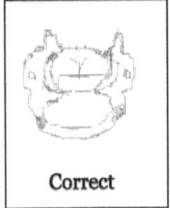

| Too Large | Too Small | Correct |

Select a clamp that will maintain four -point contact
 with the tooth's proximal
surface .If a clamp is too large , it will impringe on the soft tissue .
If it is too smalll
, it will not properly grasp the tooth surface and will be unstable

Clamps Types

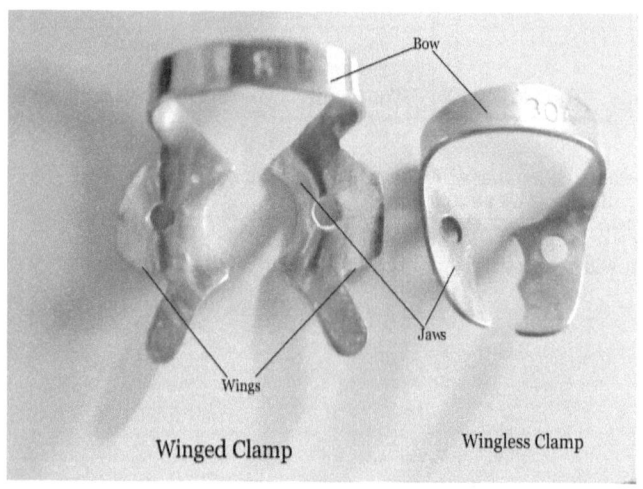

Bow

Jaws

Wings

Winged Clamp

Wingless Clamp

Dental Dam Forceps:

They utilize for placement and removal of the retainers or clamps.

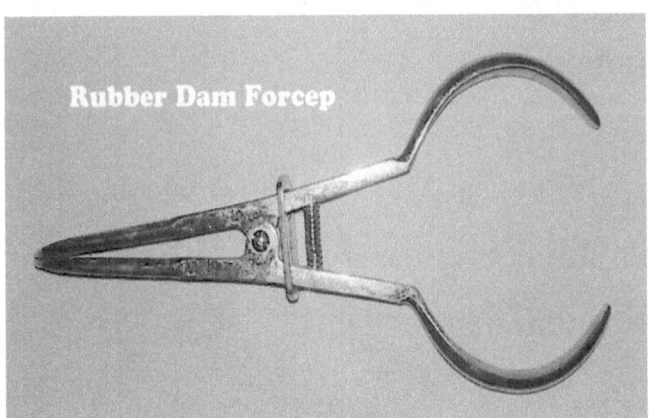

Rubber Dam Forcep

Rubber Dam Punch :

Having holes of varying sizes .The plunger
must be centered in the cutting hole ;in that,
the edges of the holes are not at risk of being
chipped when the plunger is closed.
Otherwise , the cutting quality of the punch
is ruined.

My Method is Marking the position of the
teeth directly in the mouth using a
Permanent marker

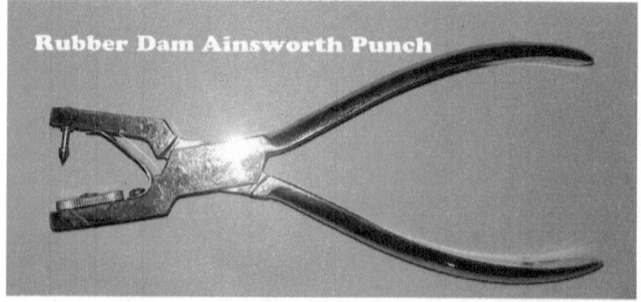

Rubber Dam Frame :

Rubber dam frame supports the edge of
Rubber Dam .

It retracts the soft tissue .

It improves accessibility of the isolated teeth
.

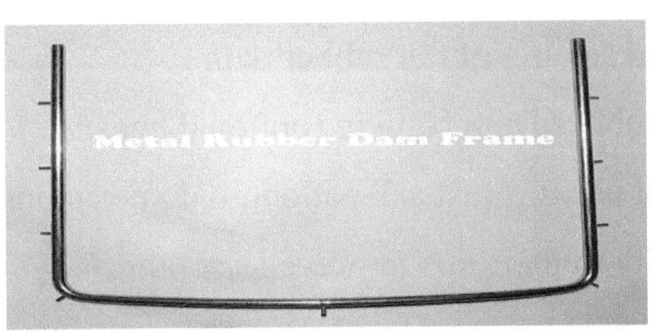

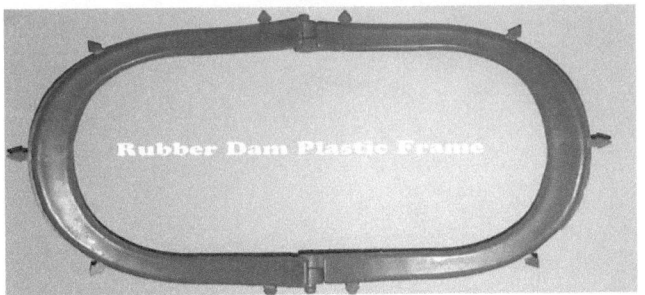

Rubber Dam accessories:

-Lubricant/petroleum jelly / shaving cream :Applying the lubricant to both sides of the dam in the area of the punched holes to assist in passing the dam through the contacts .

-Dental floss or Teflon Tape for inversion and sealing of the rubber dam .

-Rubber Dam Napkin (optional because I do not use it .I just ask patient to do petroleum jelly to their lips to prevent irritation) .

Anchors :

Other anchors beside the clamps are waxed

dental floss or small piece of rubber dam or rubber wedjet which I always prefer which is passed through the proximal contact.
See photos below .

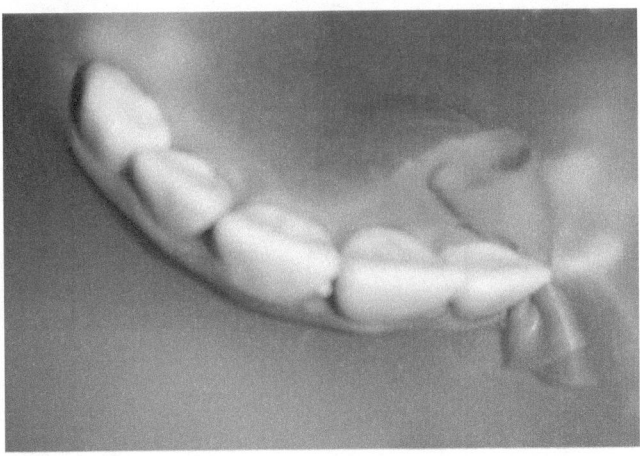

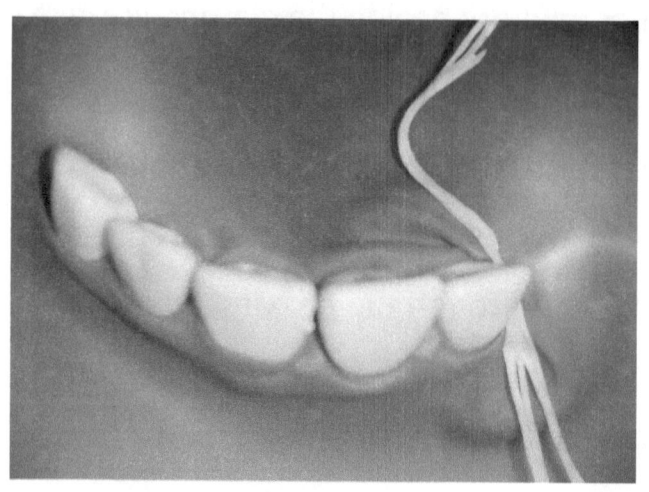

Hole size and Position :

Most punches of the rubber dam have either five or six holes .
The smallers holes for the incisors ,canines and premolars .The larger holes for the molars .

Punch Table

#5 Anchor Molar

#4 Molars

#3 Bicuspids & Canines

#2 Maxillary Anterior Incisors
#1 Mandibular Anterior Incisors

Isolation Field :

Identify which teeth to isolate
Isolation field can be the following :
Posterior Isolation
Anterior Isolation
Single tooth Isolation
Pediatric Isolation.

In general ,single isolation is done when you have class I , v fillings or endodontic treatment.While multiple isolation is required when you have class II or quardant dentistry or bleaching.

See the following photos .

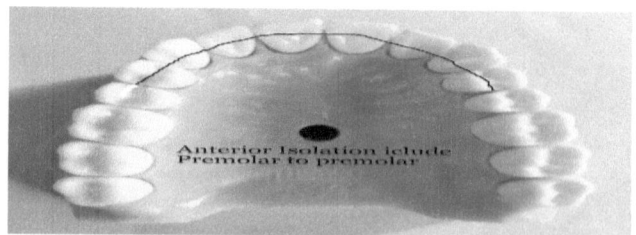

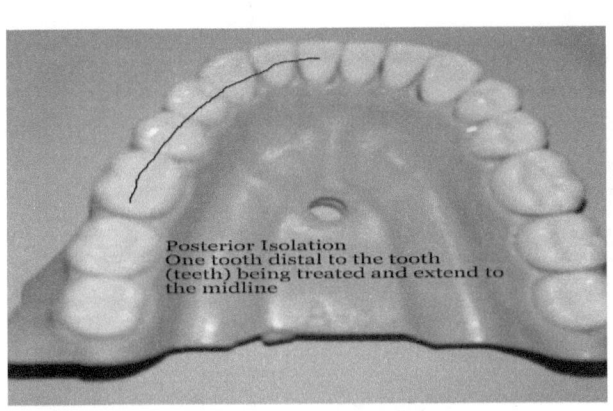

Posterior Isolation
One tooth distal to the tooth
(teeth) being treated and extend to
the midline

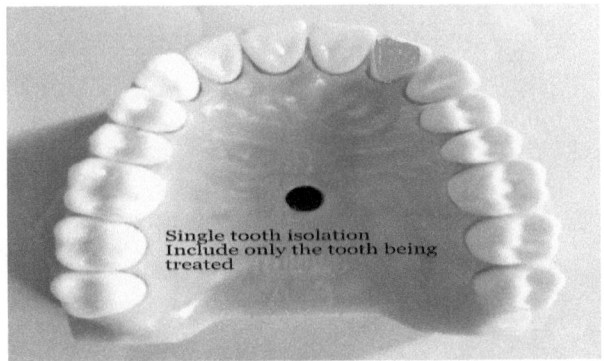

Single tooth isolation
Include only the tooth being
treated

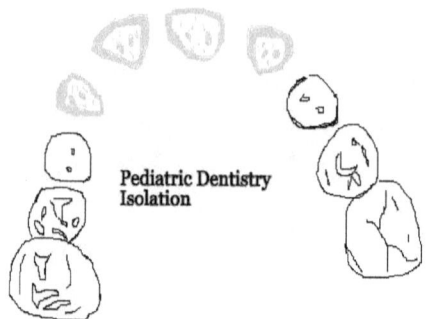

Pediatric Dentistry
Isolation

Isolate one tooth mesial and distal to the tooth (teeth) being treated

Rubber Dam Template :

It is an inked rubber stamp which helps in marking dots on the sheet according to the position of the teeth.

Holes must be punched according to the arch and missing teeth.

My method is simply put the dam on the teeth and mark with pen the position of the holes directly in the mouth.

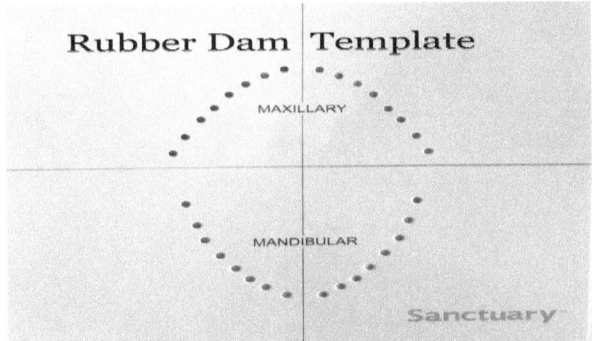

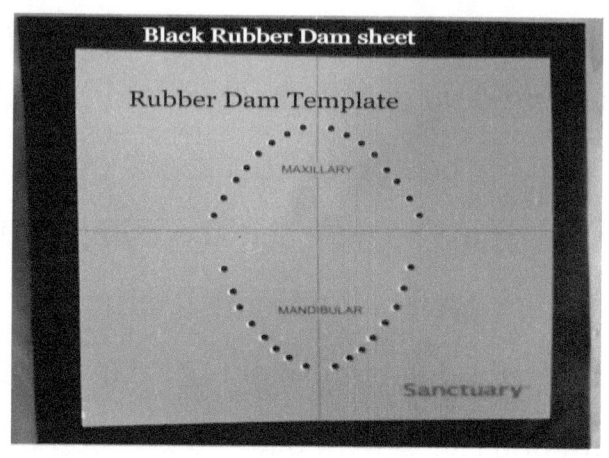

Black Rubber Dam sheet

Technique of Rubber Dam Placement

Technique 1:

Clamp Placed before rubber dam :

In patient mouth Anesthesia must be assessed ,lubricate the dam from both sides. Lubricate the lip with the corners of the patient mouth. Use dental floss to remove the debris from interproximal area .

Select the appropriate clamp according to the tooth size .

You can tie a floss to the clamp bow and place the clamp onto the tooth .

Larger holes are required in this technique
since the rubber needs to be stretched over
the clamp usually two or three overlapping
holes are made .

Stretch the rubber dam over the clamp

See photos below

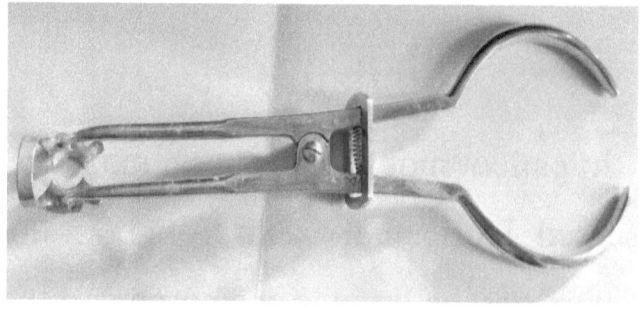

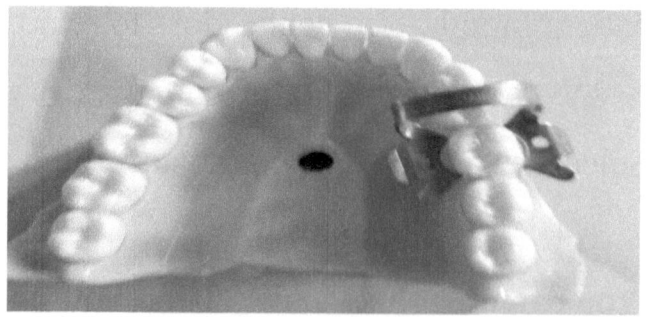

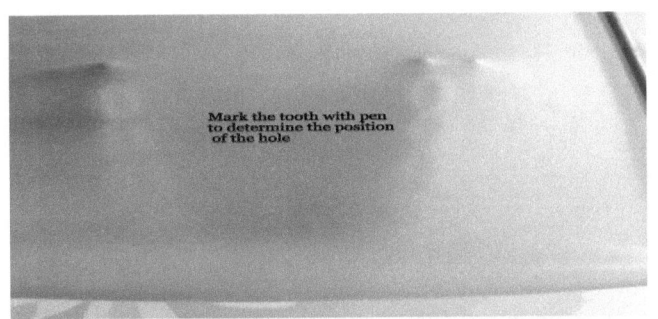

Mark the tooth with pen
to determine the position
of the hole

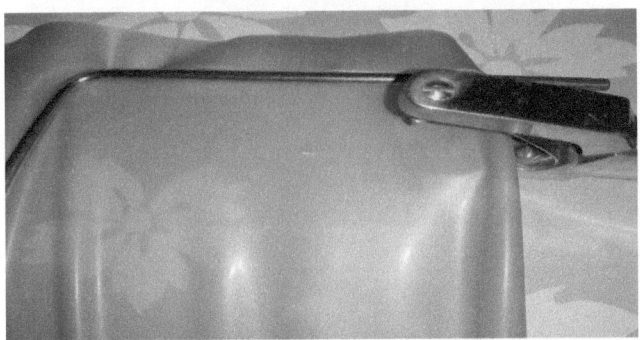

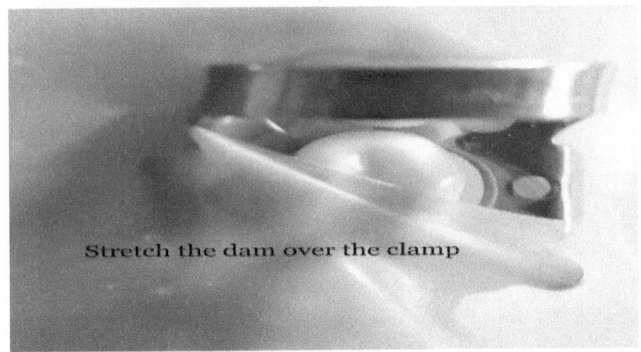

Stretch the dam over the clamp

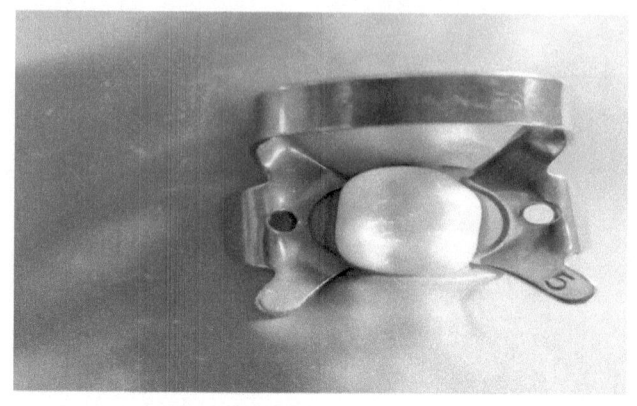

Technique 2

Placement of the rubber dam and clamp together

Select the appropriate clamp.

Punch the hole in rubber dam sheet.

Clamp is held with clamp forceps and inserted into the punch hole.

Carry both the clamp and rubber dam over the crown and seat it.

Remove the forceps from the clamp .

Release the rubber dam from the wings to lie around the cervical margin of the tooth .

See the following photos .

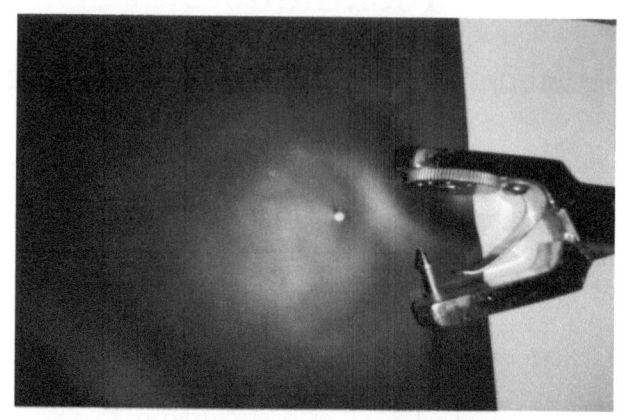

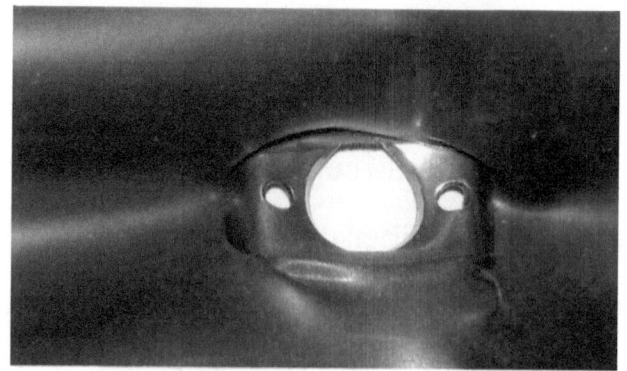

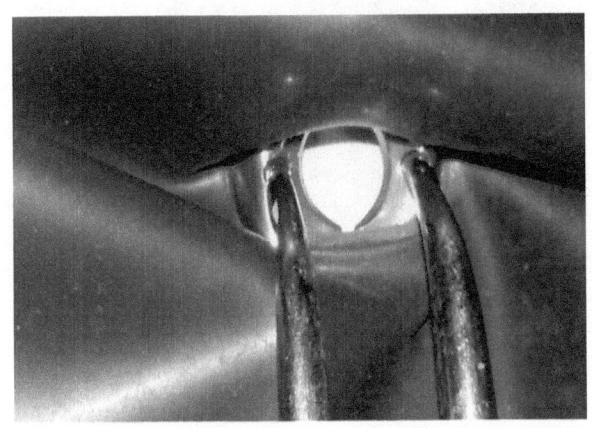

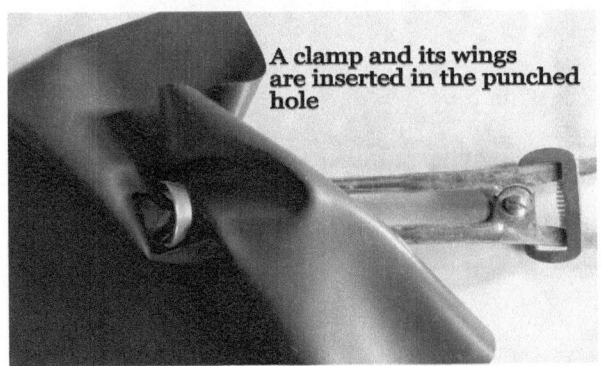

A clamp and its wings are inserted in the punched hole

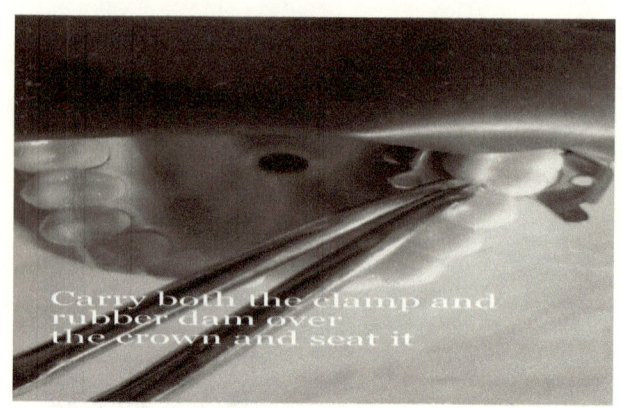

Carry both the clamp and rubber dam over the crown and seat it

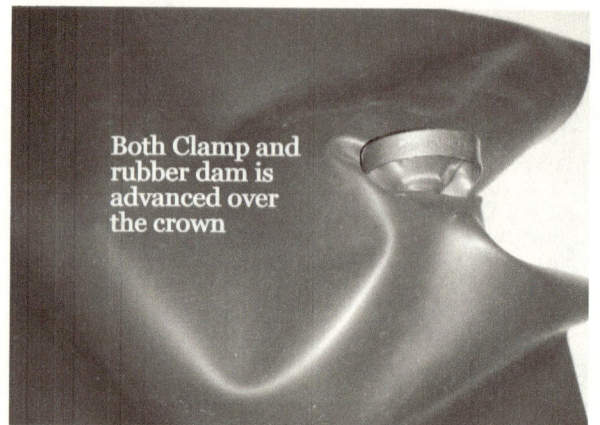

Both Clamp and rubber dam is advanced over the crown

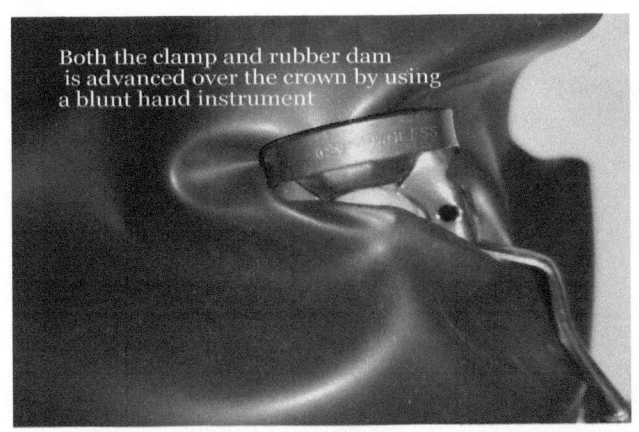

Both the clamp and rubber dam is advanced over the crown by using a blunt hand instrument

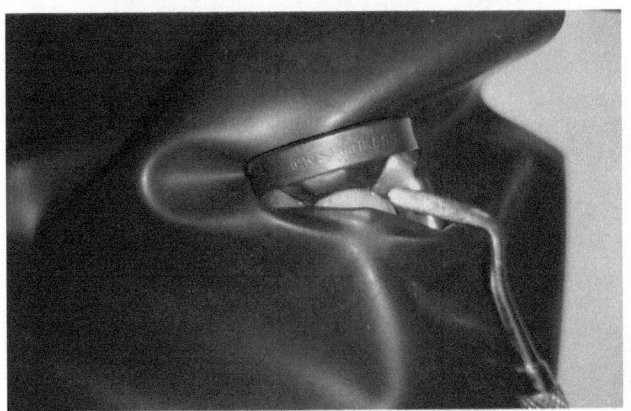

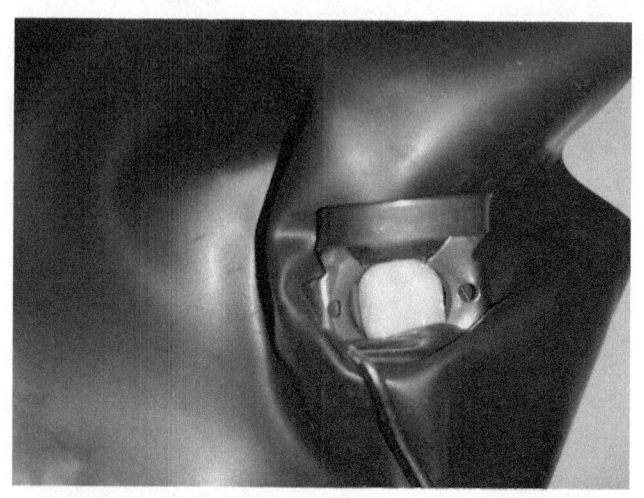

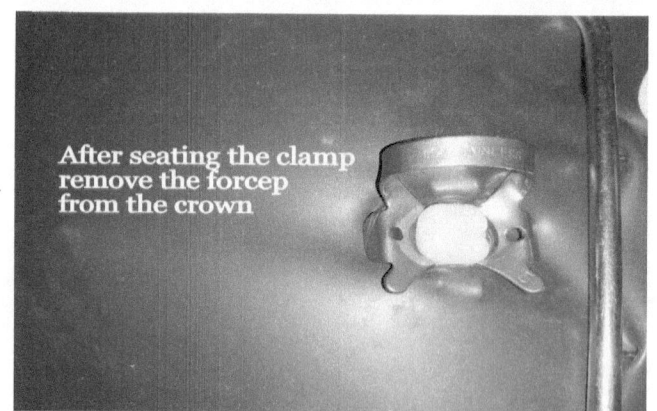

After seating the clamp
remove the forcep
from the crown

Technique 3
Split Dam Technique

In this method the rubber dam is used and placed to isolate the tooth without clamp. In this method , two overlapping holes are punched in the dam .Then, dam is stretched over the tooth to be treated and over the adjacent teeth on each side .Edge of the rubber dam is carefully teased through the contact of the adjacent teeth in the distal side.

It is utilized to isolate anterior teeth .Also, when there is insufficient crown structure. Moreover, it used when isolate teeth with porcelain crowns because the

clamp can damage the cervical porcelain.

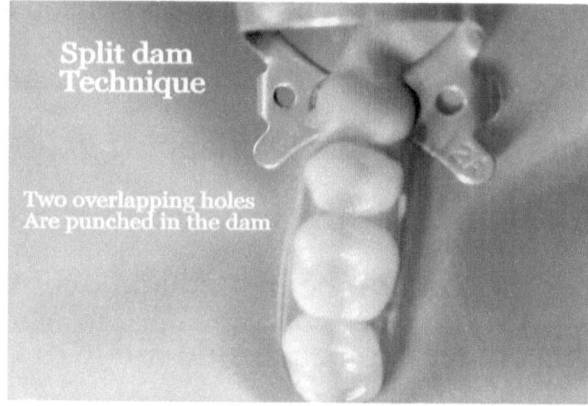

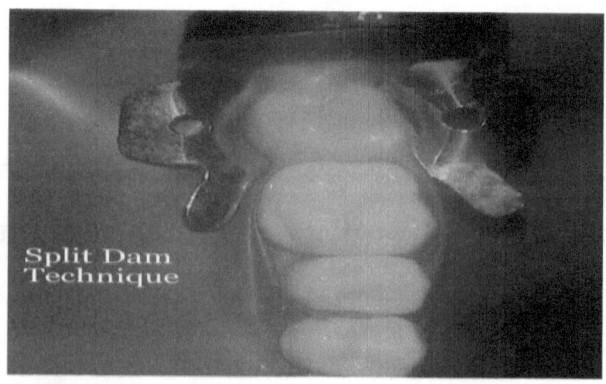

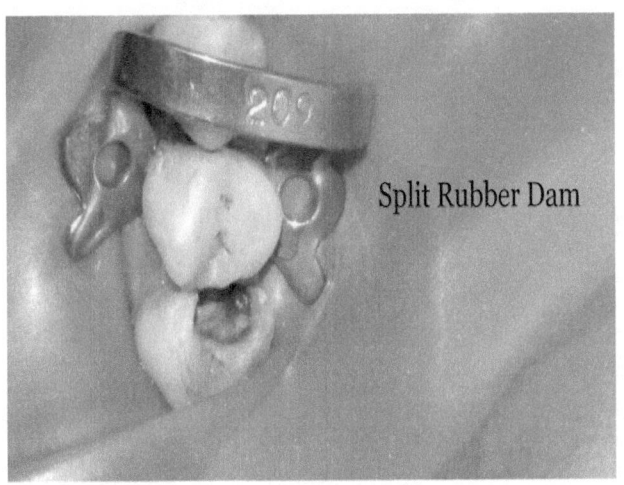

Split Rubber Dam

Sleeve Rubber Dam Technique

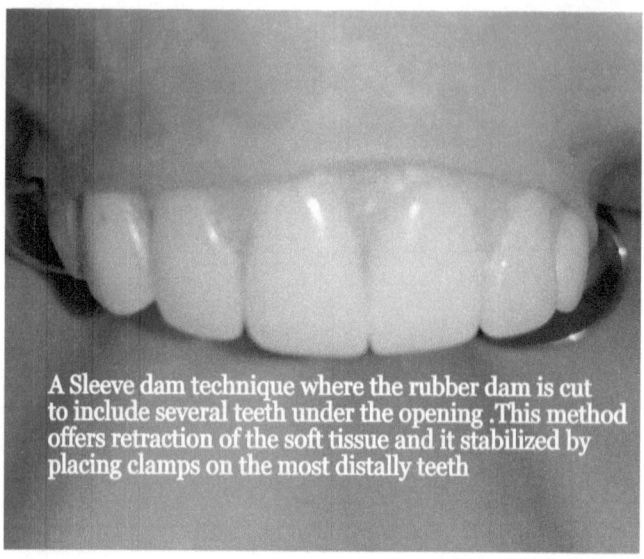

A Sleeve dam technique where the rubber dam is cut to include several teeth under the opening .This method offers retraction of the soft tissue and it stabilized by placing clamps on the most distally teeth

Leakage:

Sometimes when you isolate single tooth
or multiple teeth leakage is seen through
the rubber dam .You can seal this leakage
by using temporary filling material,
periodontal packs, or liquid Rubber
dam .But, if the gaps is large , rubber
dam must be replaced .

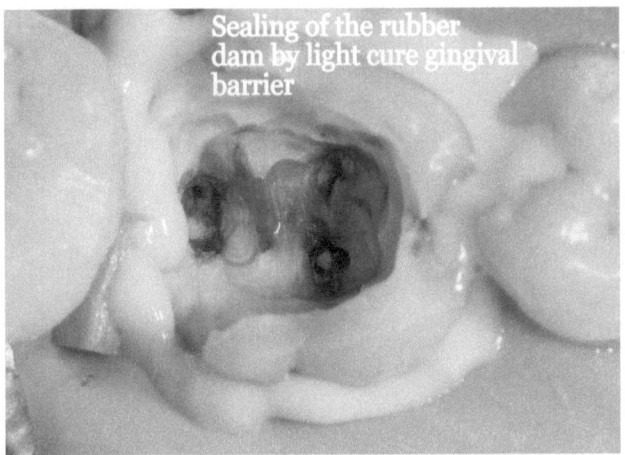

Sealing of the rubber
dam by light cure gingival
barrier

Removal Of Rubber Dam :

Use the clamp forcep to remove the clamp before cutting the dam or after. Before the rubber dam is removed , use the saliva ejector to flush out all debris .Cut away away the tied thread from the neck of the teeth if you utilize the dental floss. Stretch the dam and pull the septal rubber dam away from the gingival tissue and cut the dam with scissor . After Removing the rubber dam check with dental floss if there are missing pieces of rubber .

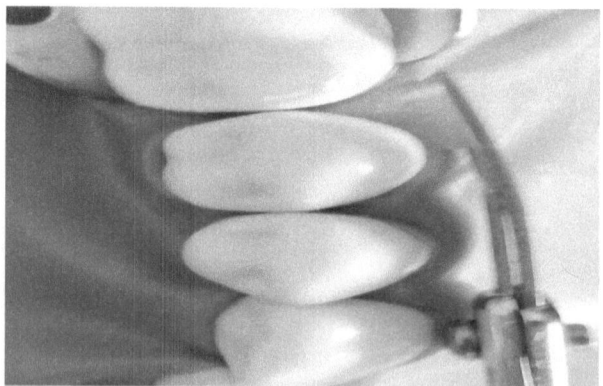

Method Of Tying clamp with dental floss:

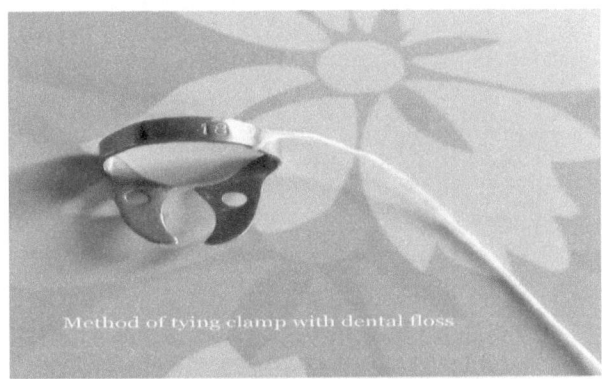

Method of tying clamp with dental floss

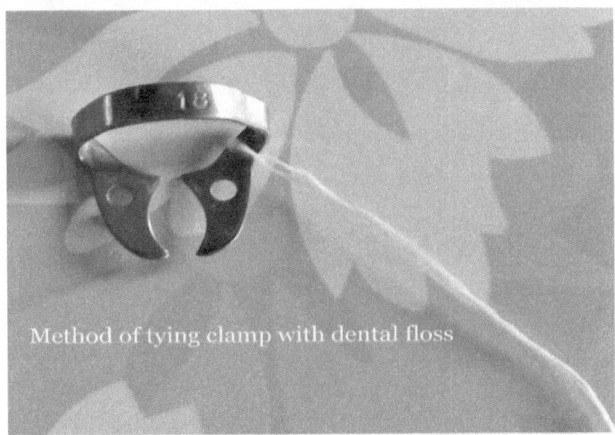

Method of tying clamp with dental floss

Examples of Isolation Of Teeth :

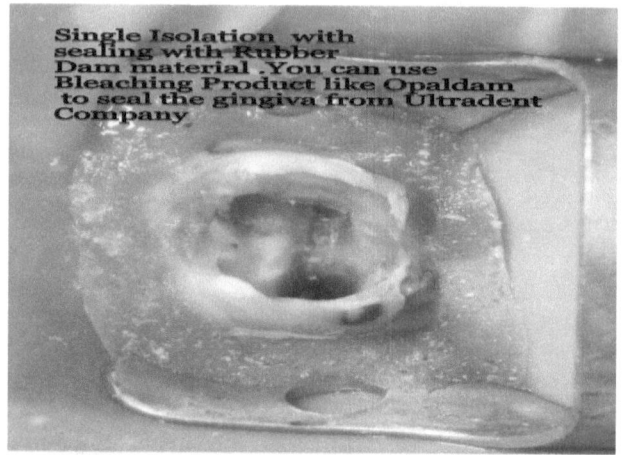

Single Isolation with sealing with Rubber Dam material . You can use Bleaching Product like Opaldam to seal the gingiva from Ultradent Company

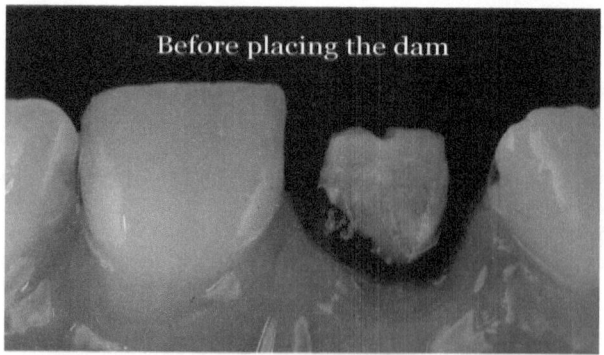

Before placing the dam

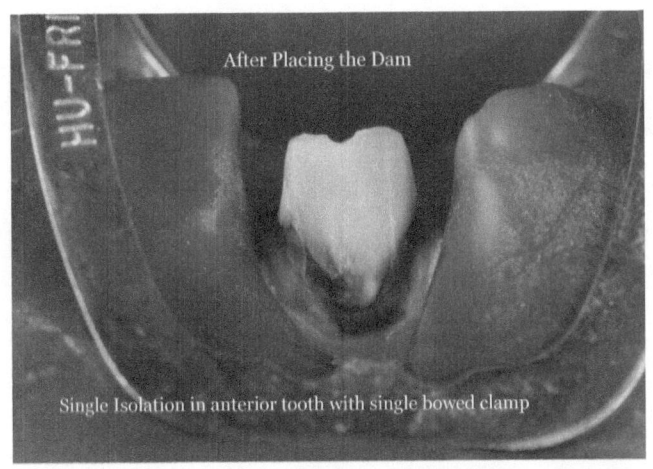

After Placing the Dam

Single Isolation in anterior tooth with single bowed clamp

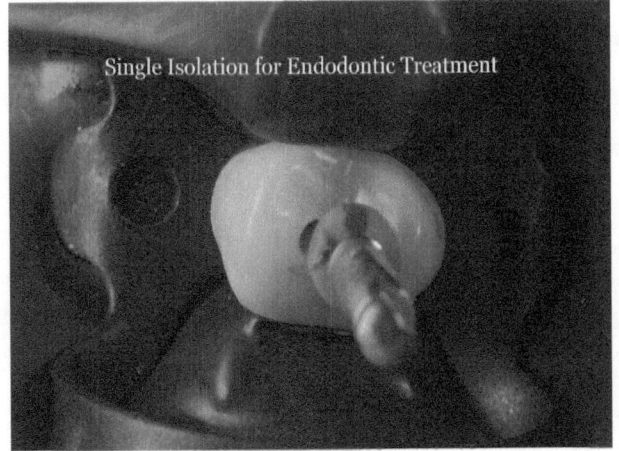

Single Isolation for Endodontic Treatment

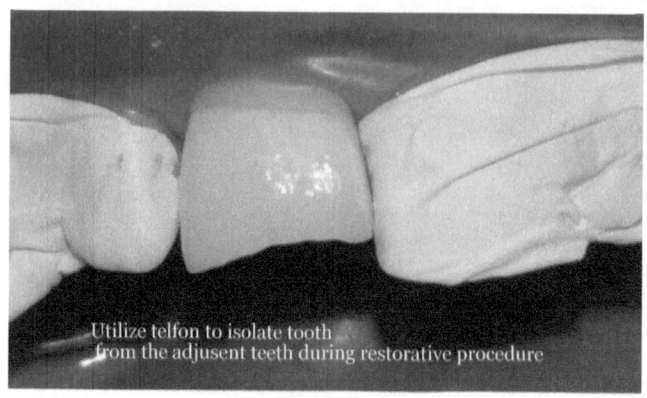

Utilize telfon to isolate tooth
from the adjusent teeth during restorative procedure

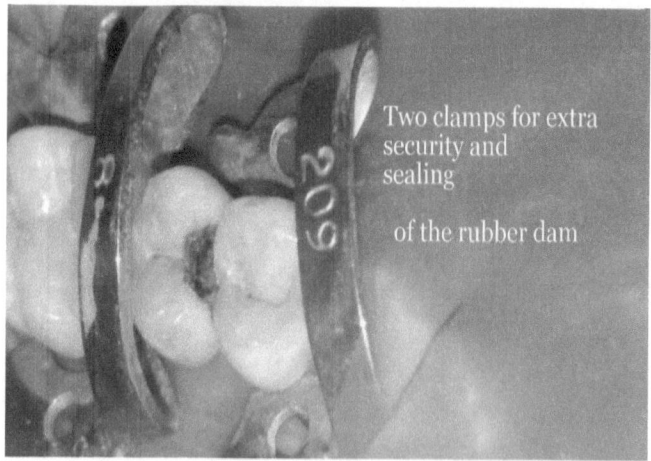

Two clamps for extra
security and
sealing

of the rubber dam

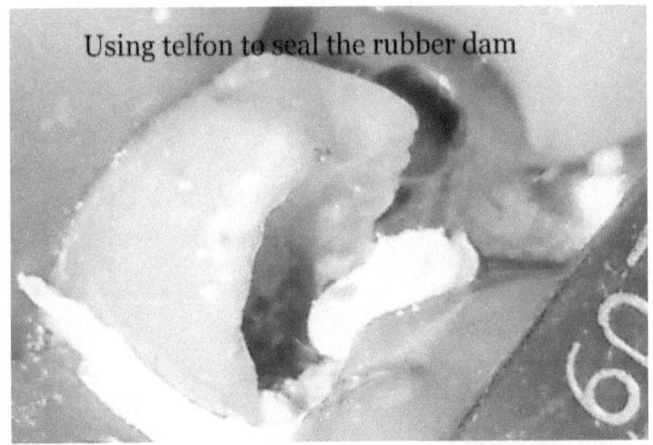

Using telfon to seal the rubber dam

Dr.Calogero 's Case

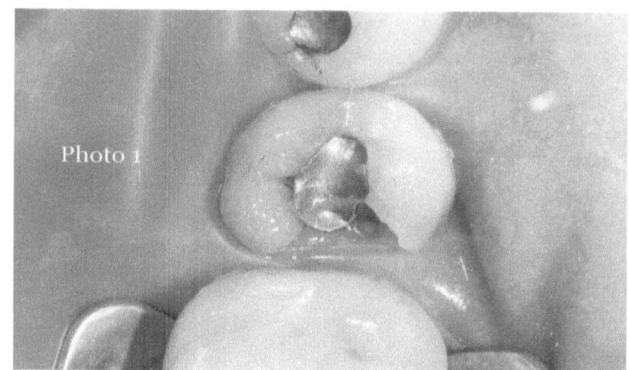

Photo 1

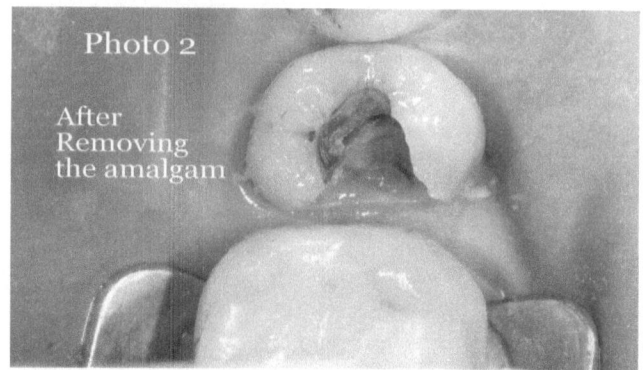

Photo 2

After
Removing
the amalgam

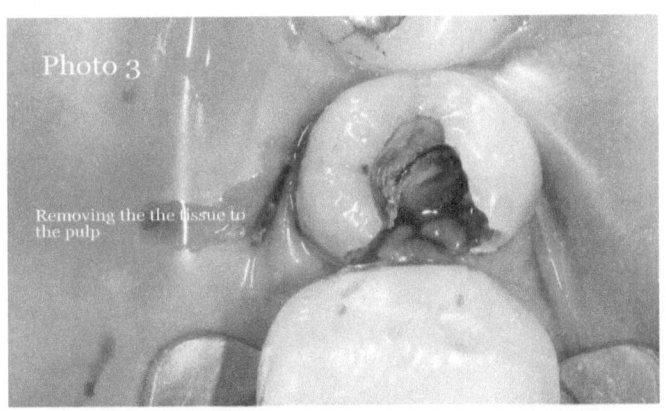

Photo 3

Removing the the tissue to the pulp

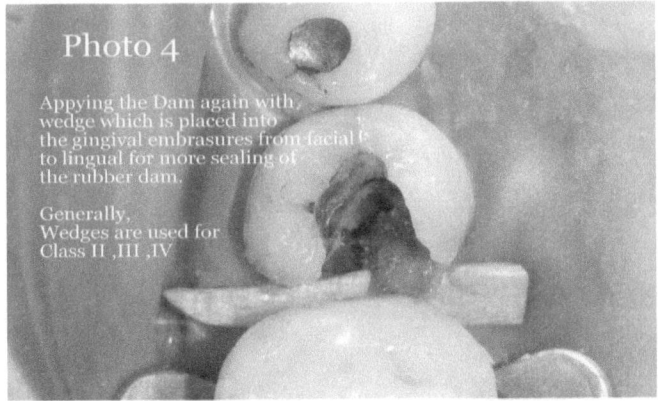

Photo 4

Appying the Dam again with wedge which is placed into the gingival embrasures from facial to lingual for more sealing of the rubber dam.

Generally, Wedges are used for Class II ,III ,IV

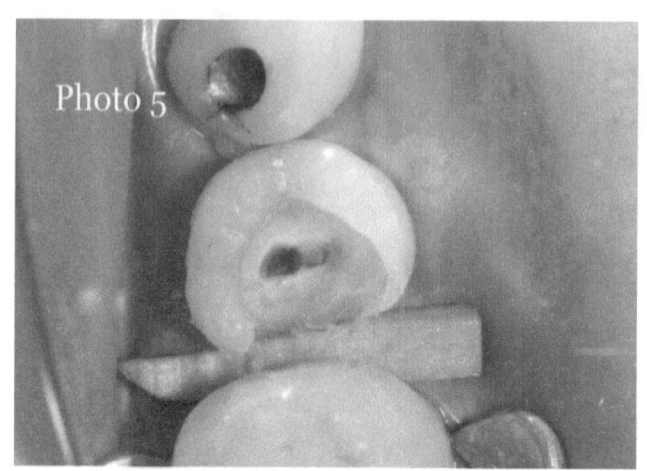

Photo 5

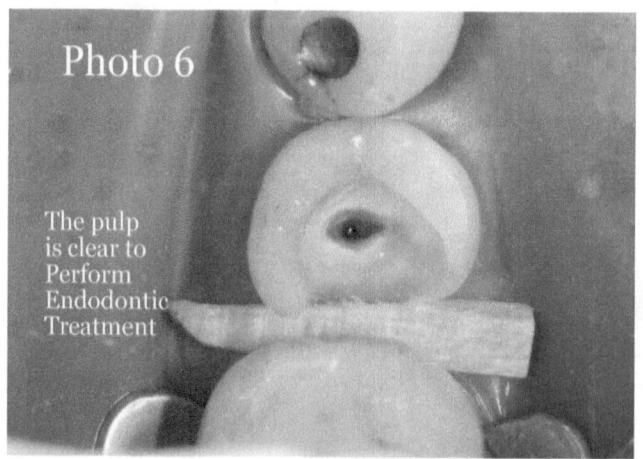

Photo 6

The pulp
is clear to
Perform
Endodontic
Treatment

Another Case of Dr.Calogero

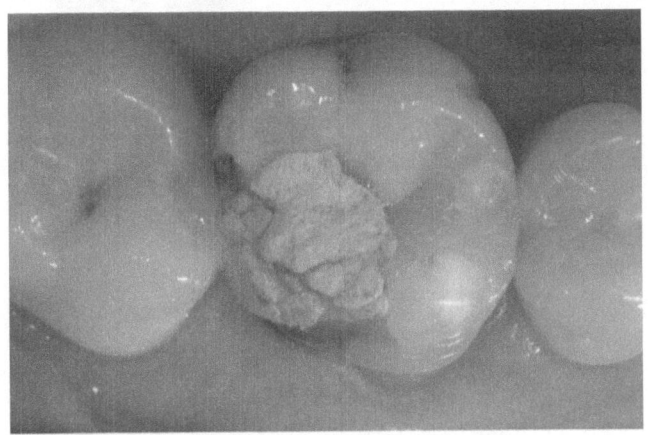

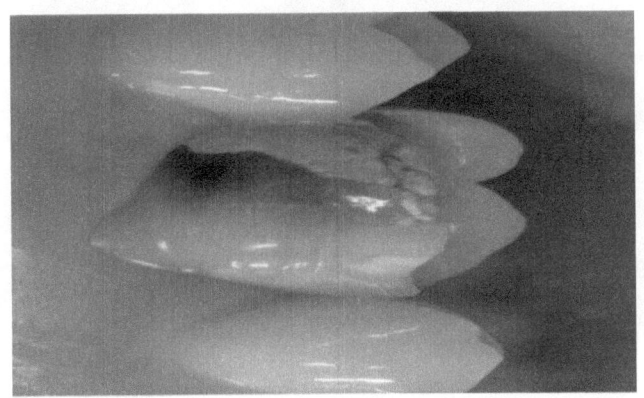

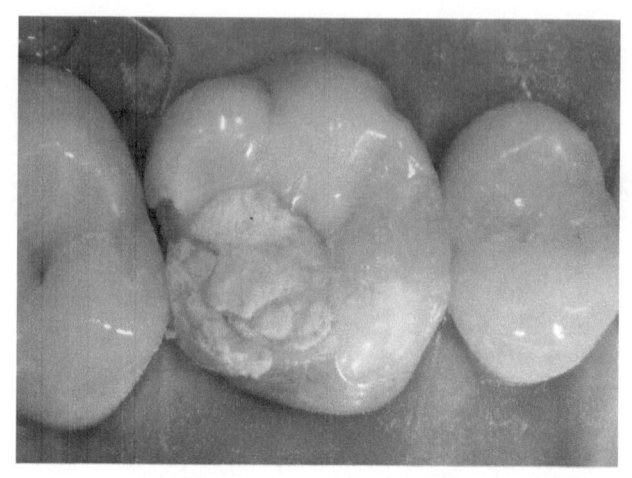

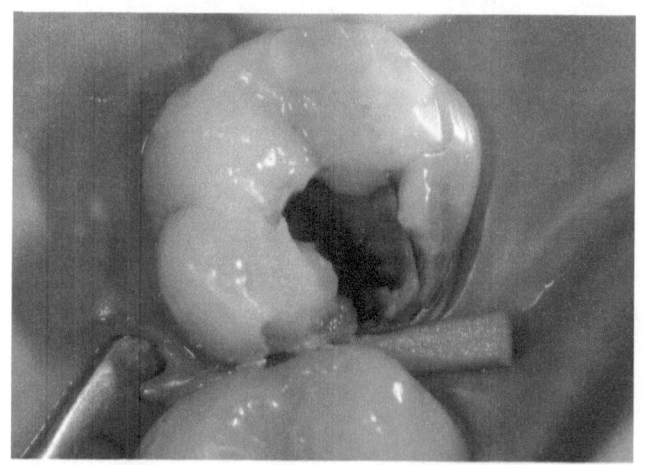

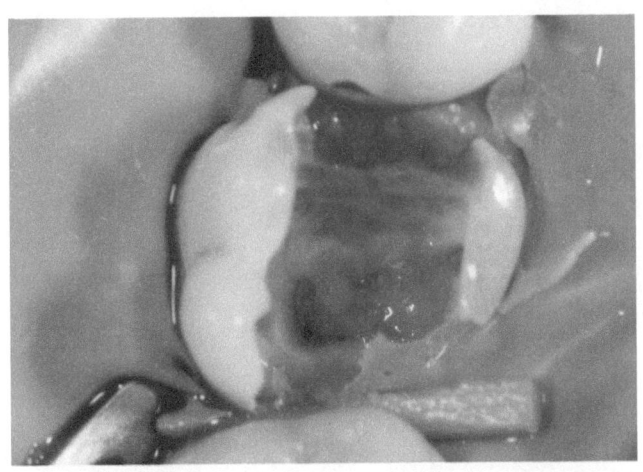

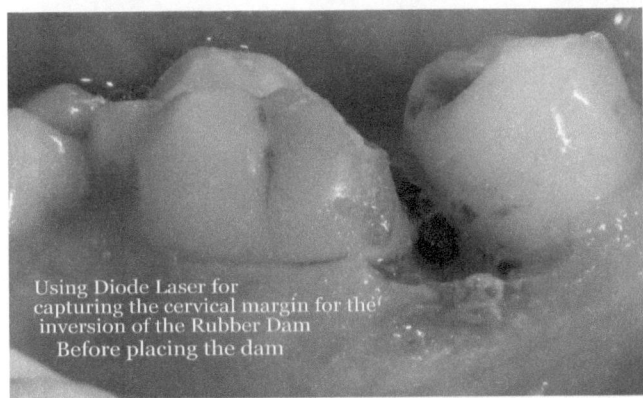

Using Diode Laser for
capturing the cervical margin for the
inversion of the Rubber Dam
Before placing the dam

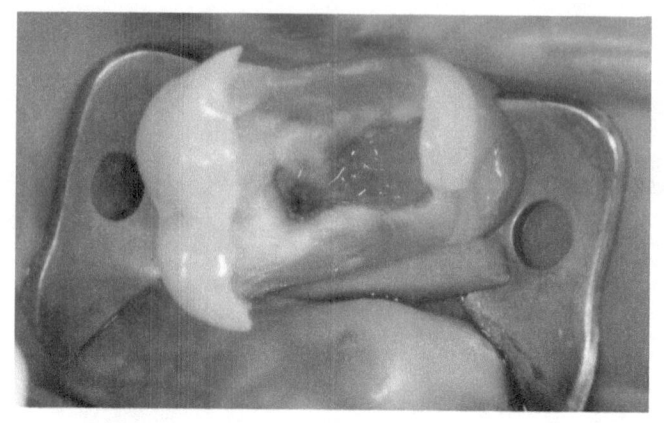

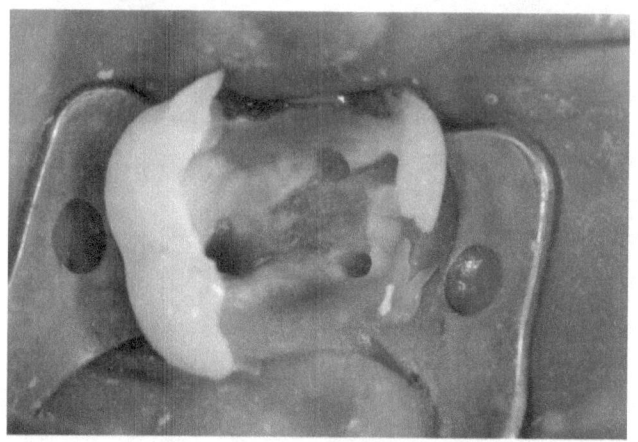

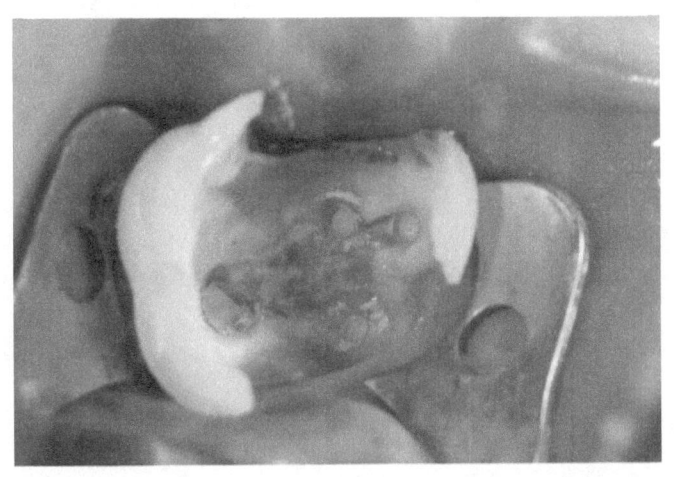

More Example of Isolation of the Teeth with Rubber Dam :

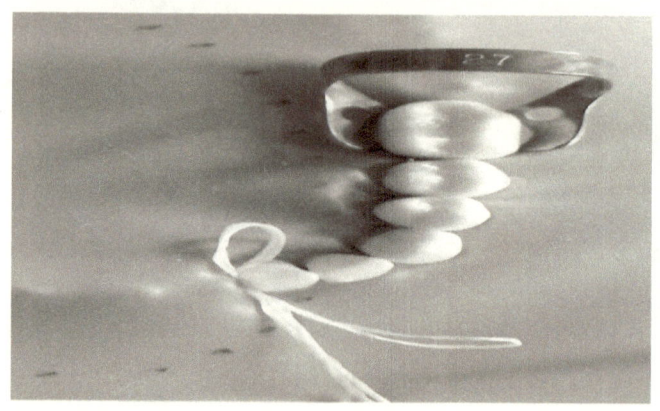

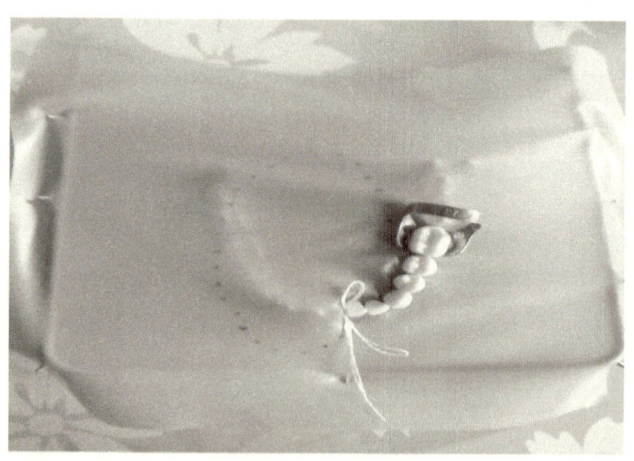

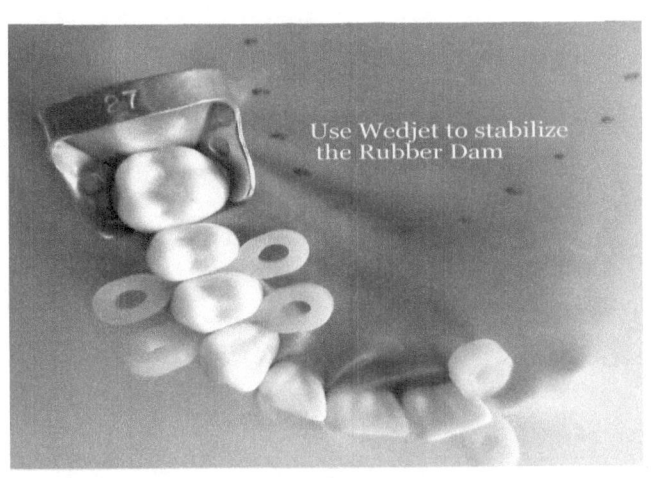

Use Wedjet to stabilize
the Rubber Dam

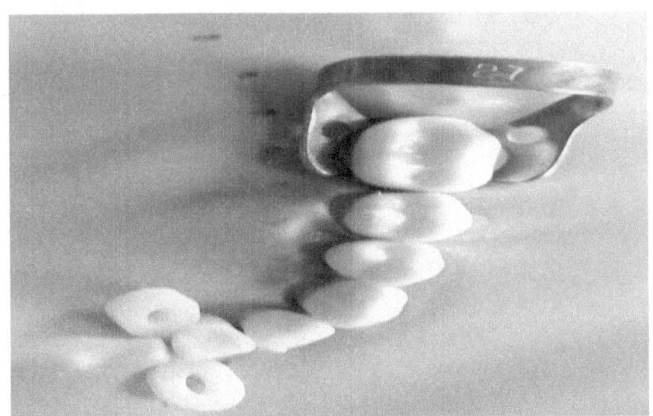

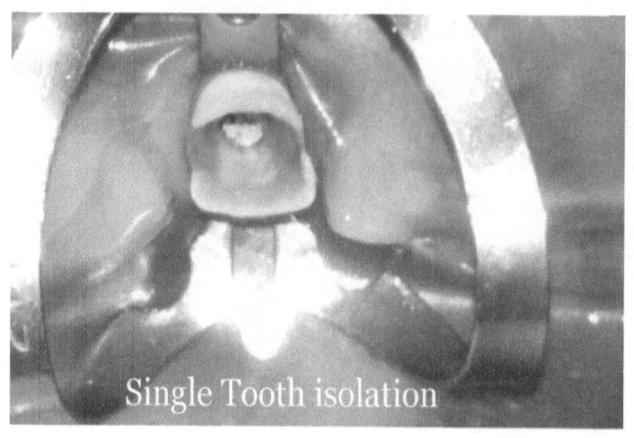

Single Tooth isolation

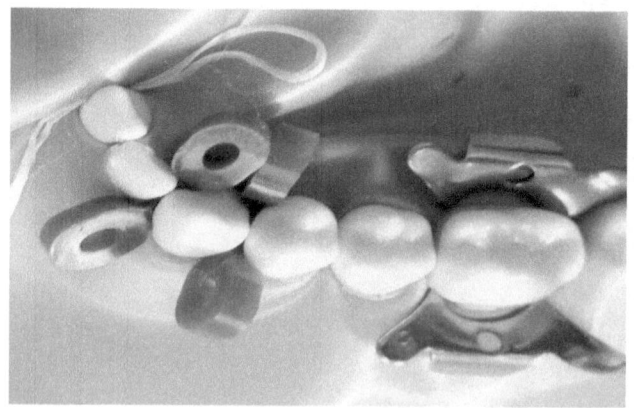

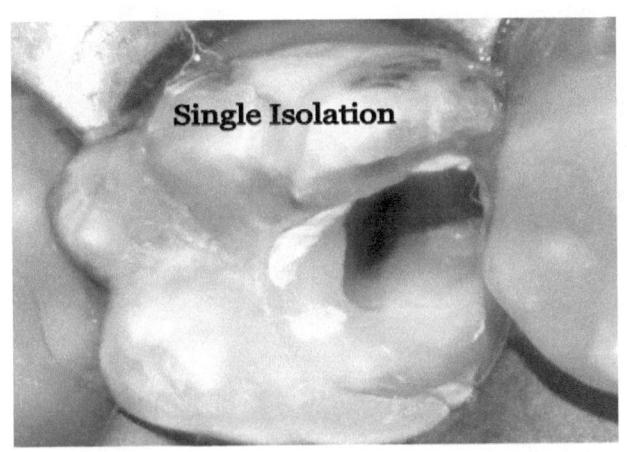

Single Isolation

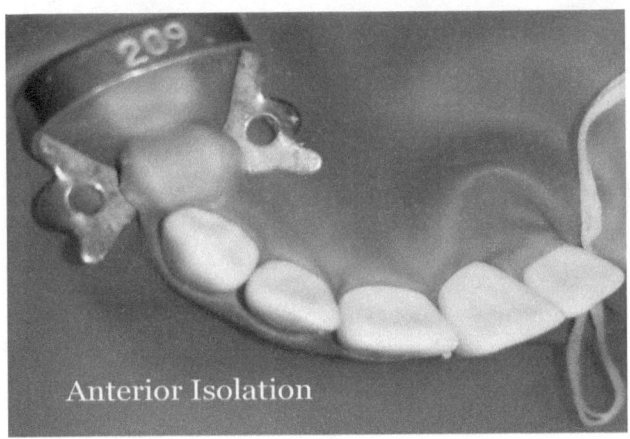

Anterior Isolation

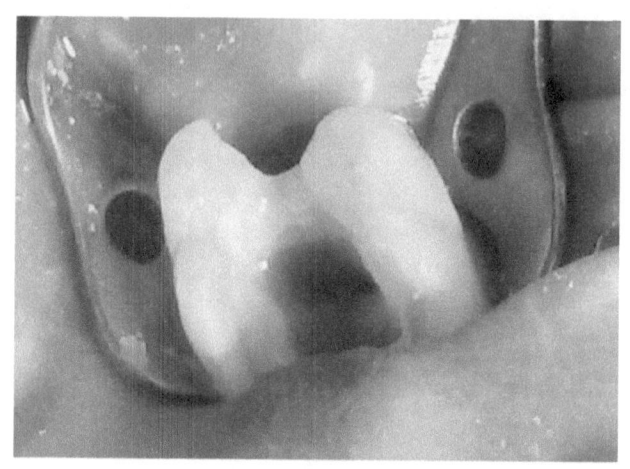

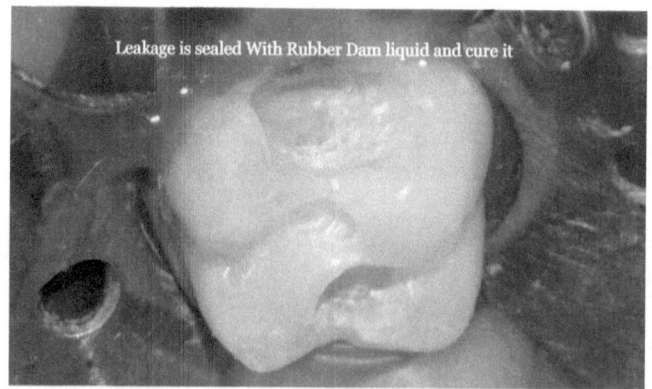

Leakage is sealed With Rubber Dam liquid and cure it

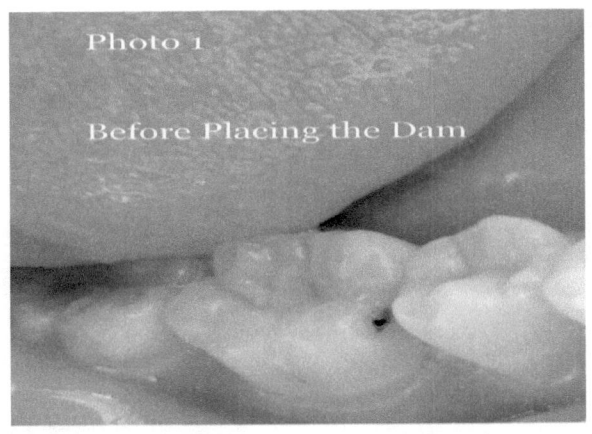

Photo 1

Before Placing the Dam

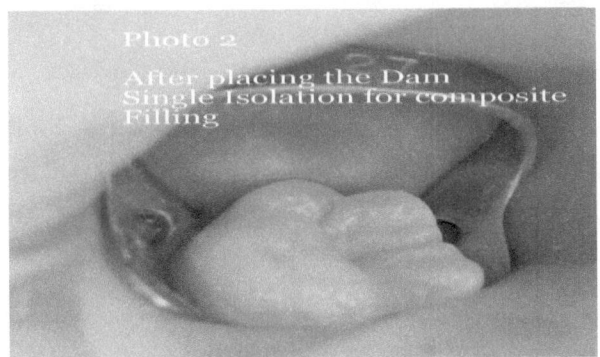

Photo 2

After placing the Dam
Single Isolation for composite
Filling

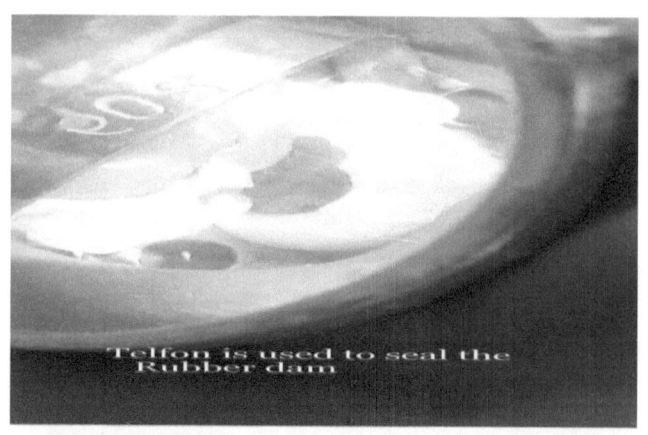

Telfon is used to seal the
Rubber dam

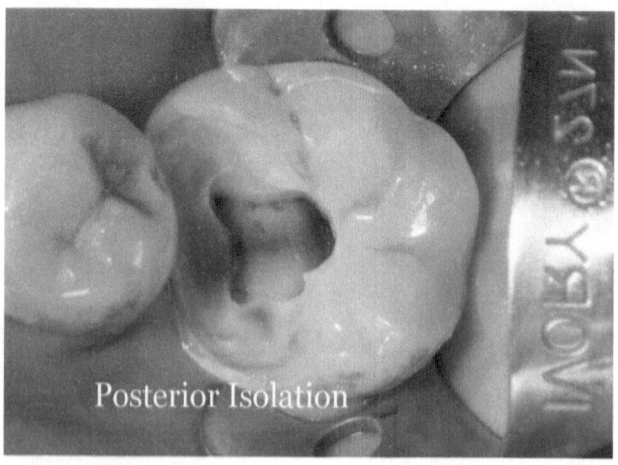

Posterior Isolation

Method of tying Dental Floss (Surgeon'sKnot):

A ,B and C, Dental Floss is placed around the tooth gingival to the height of the contour .A knot is tied by making two loops with the free ends,followed by a single loop.

E , The free ends are not cut but tied to frame to serve as a reminder that ligature is in place .**D,**Finally, to Remove the ligature, you can use scissor to cut the floss.

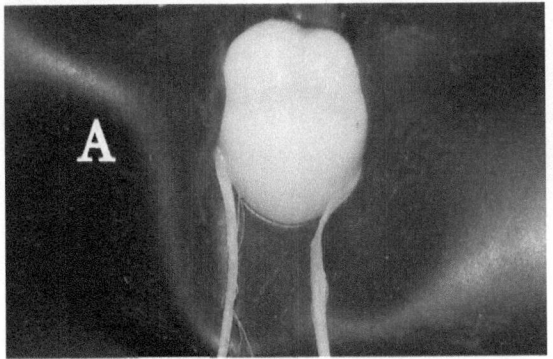

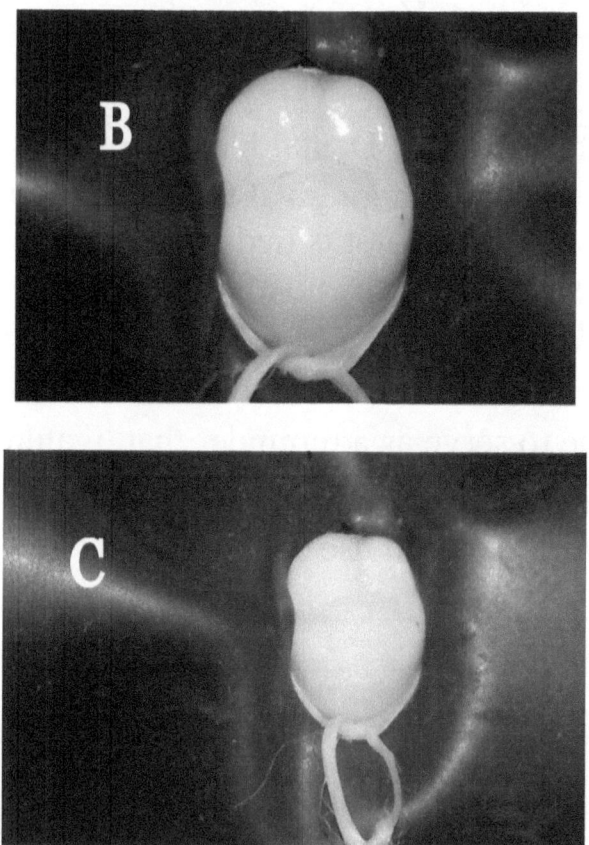

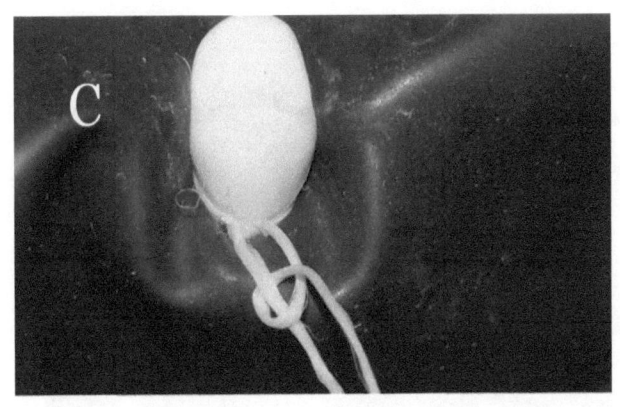

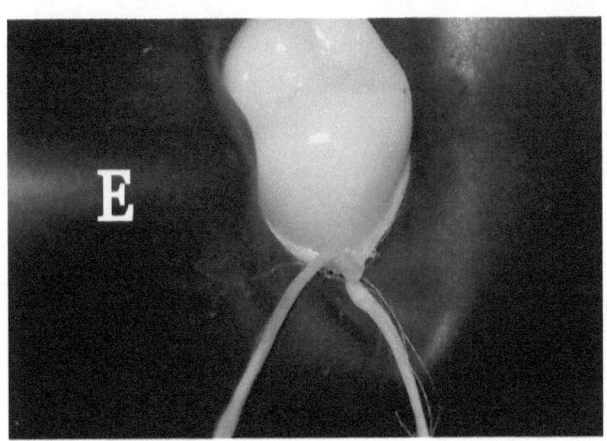

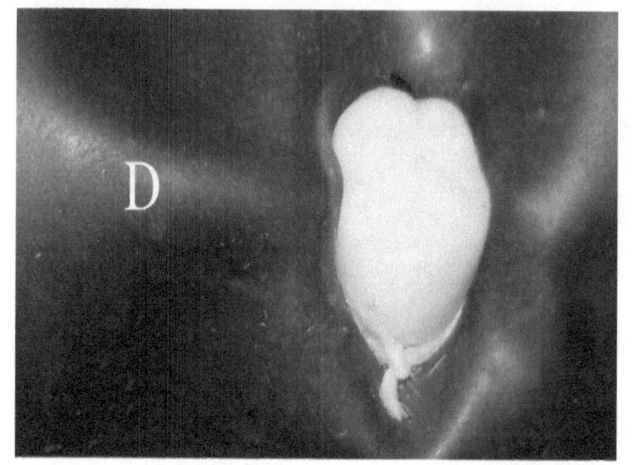

Important Tips:

- Patients with difficulty to open their mouth or they are uncomfortable to open widely , You can use a bite block with a dental floss that is attached to allow retrieval if necessary .

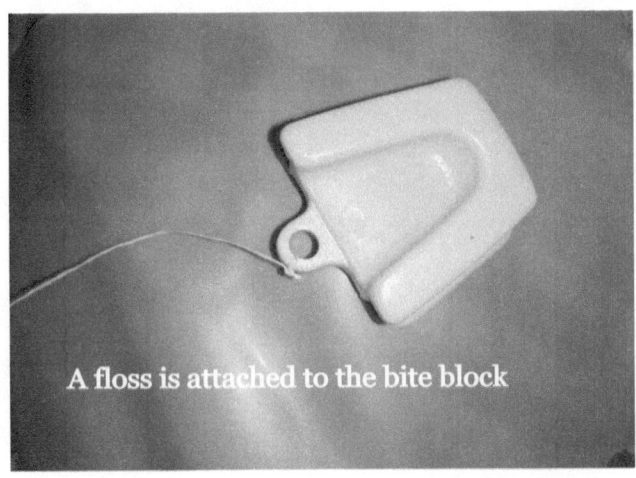

A floss is attached to the bite block

- For extra security for the rubber dam you can use more than one clamps.

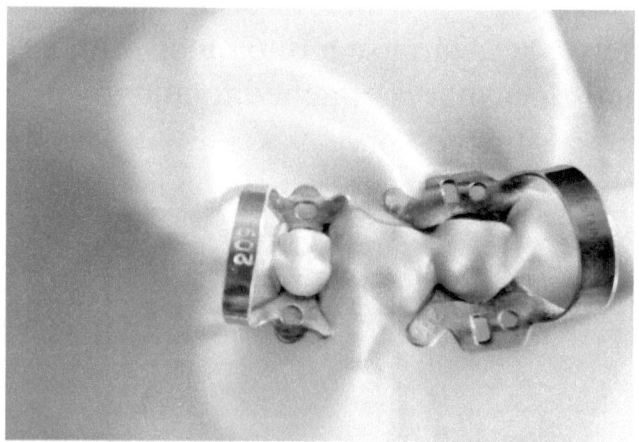

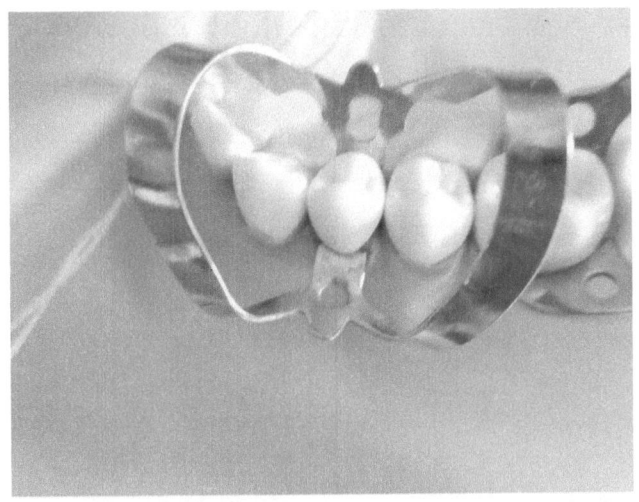

– When you utilize rubber dam
,always make a hole for the placing
of the saliva ejector through the
dam instead of placing it under the
dam. Also, protect the floor of the
mouth by placing cotton rolls or
gauze to avoid tissue injury.

- For placing single double bowed clamp .Place it first , then stretch the dam over it .

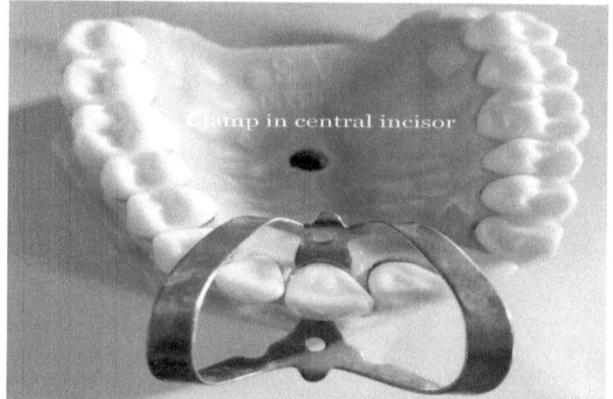

Clamp in central incisor

- Utilize dental floss to pass through the contacts for the inversion of the rubber dam interproximally. Also,using it for complete the seal around the tooth and prevent leakage. The rubber dam must be inverted towards interproximal papilla using dental floss .After moving the floss gingivally , it should be removed facially or lingually not occlusally .

See the following photos.

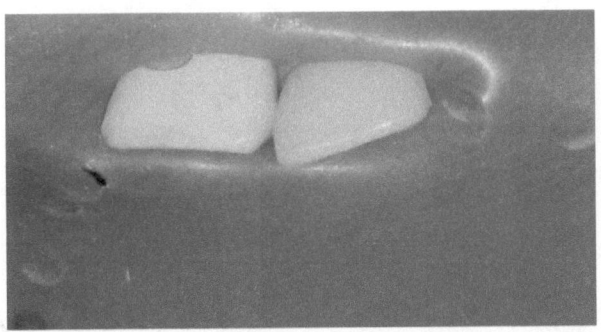

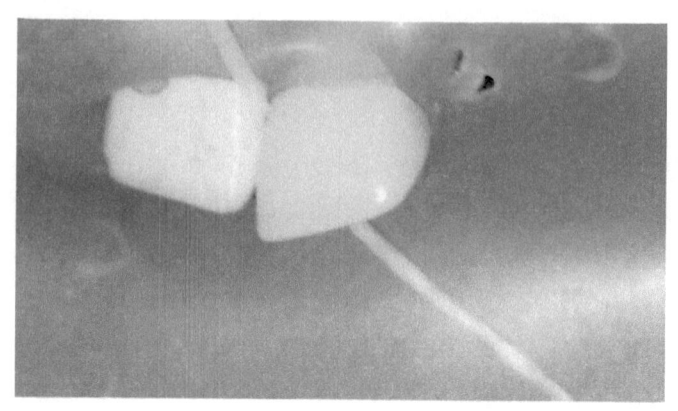

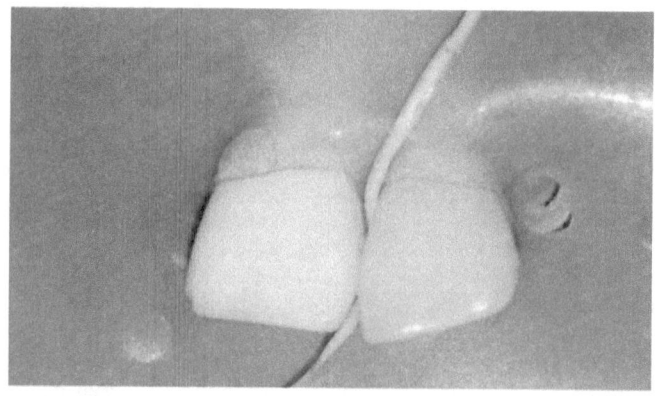

74

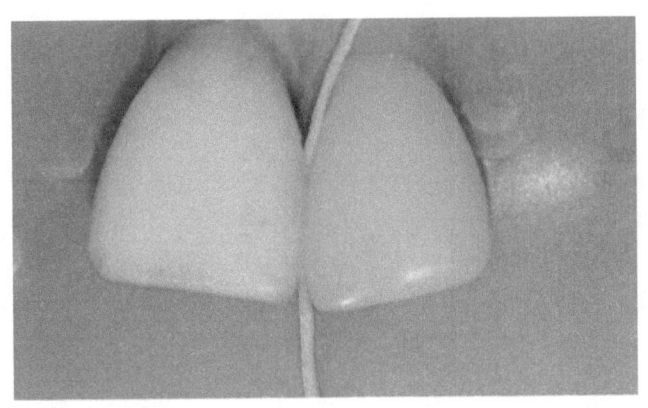

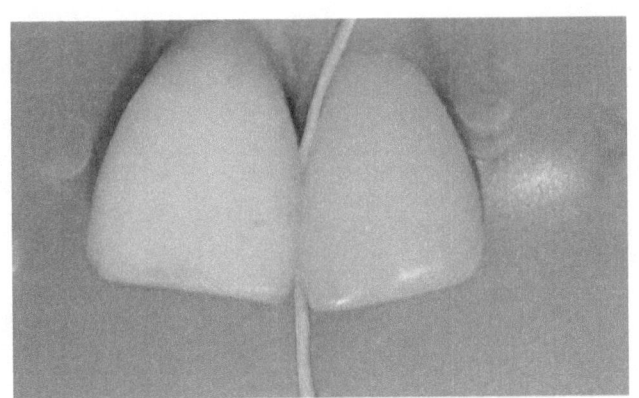

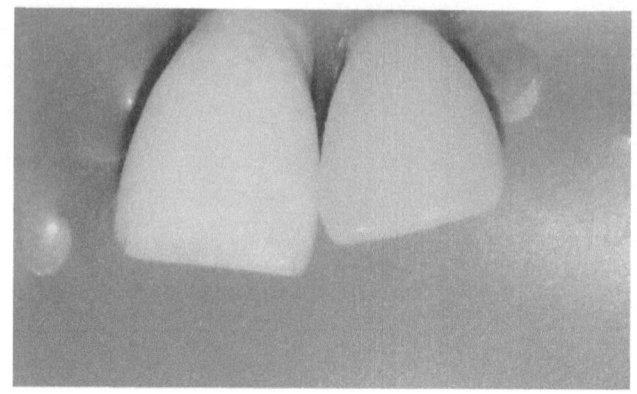

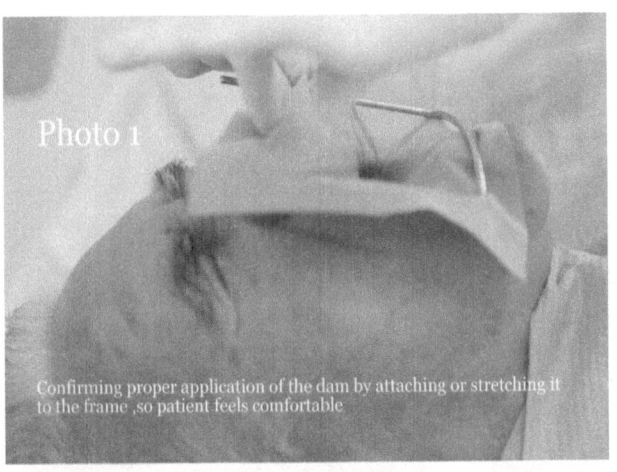

Photo 1

Confirming proper application of the dam by attaching or stretching it to the frame ,so patient feels comfortable

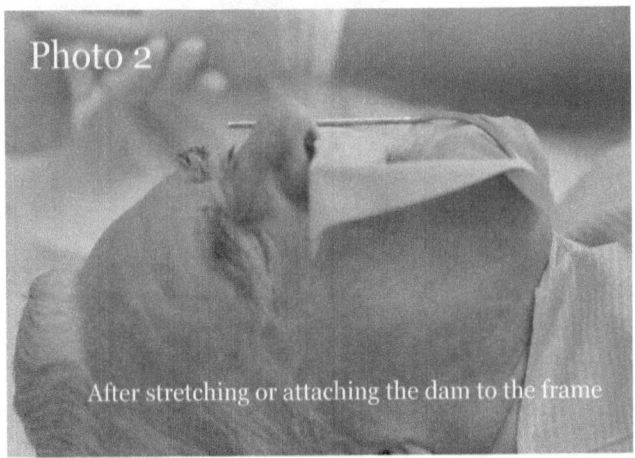

Photo 2

After stretching or attaching the dam to the frame

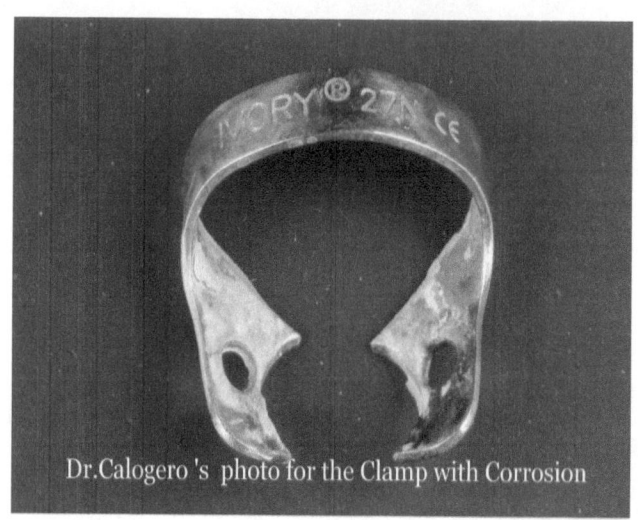

Dr.Calogero 's photo for the Clamp with Corrosion

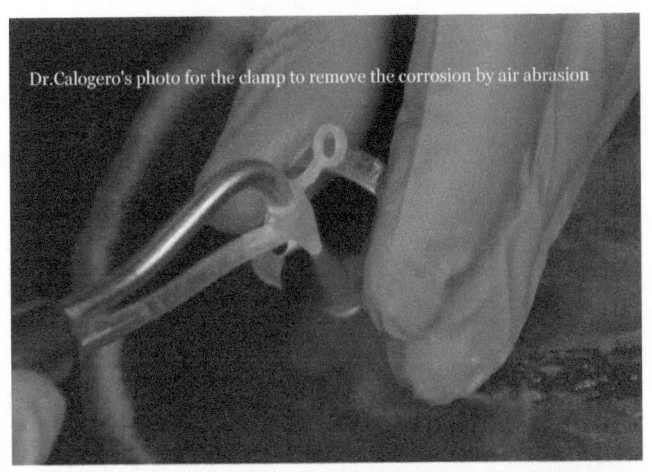

Dr.Calogero's photo for the clamp to remove the corrosion by air abrasion

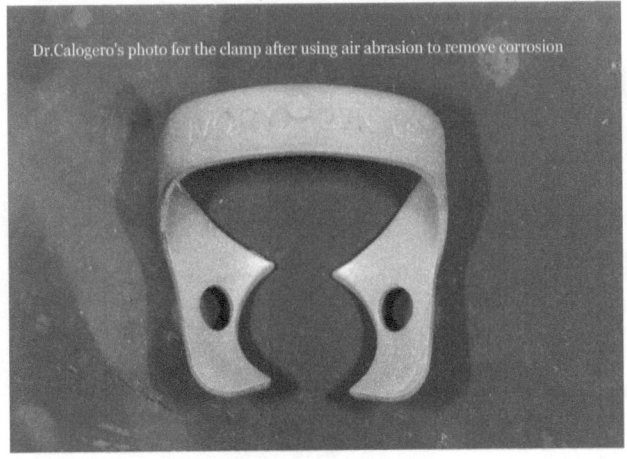

Dr.Calogero's photo for the clamp after using air abrasion to remove corrosion

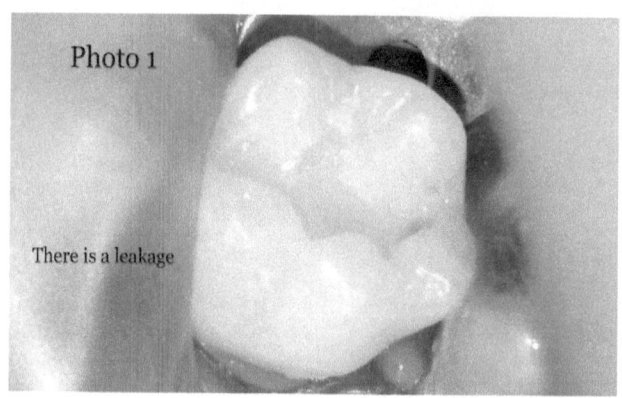

Photo 1

There is a leakage

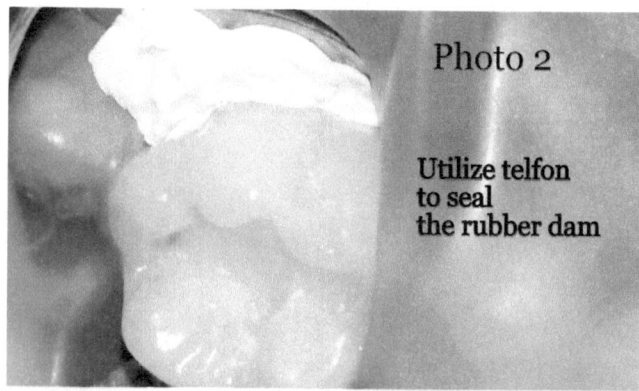

Photo 2

**Utilize telfon
to seal
the rubber dam**

- You can invert the dam facially and ligually using an explorer or blunt instrument or burnisher .Move the explorer around the tooth facially and ligually with its tip perpendicular to the tooth surface while air blowing (drying the tooth while stretching the dam gingivally and releasing it slowly).

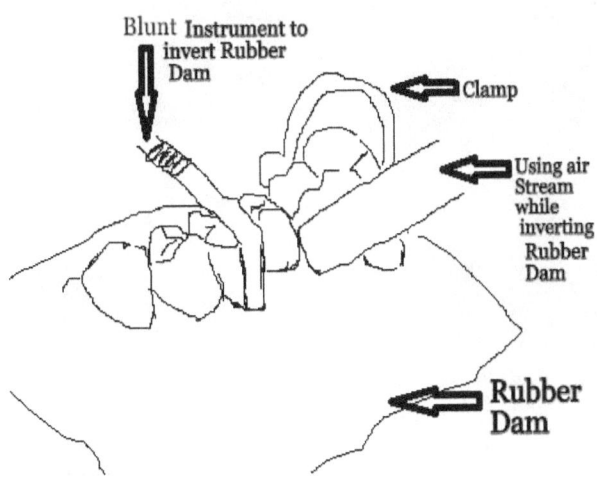

Blunt Instrument to invert Rubber Dam

Clamp

Using air Stream while inverting Rubber Dam

Rubber Dam

You see the inversion in this
anterior isolation.

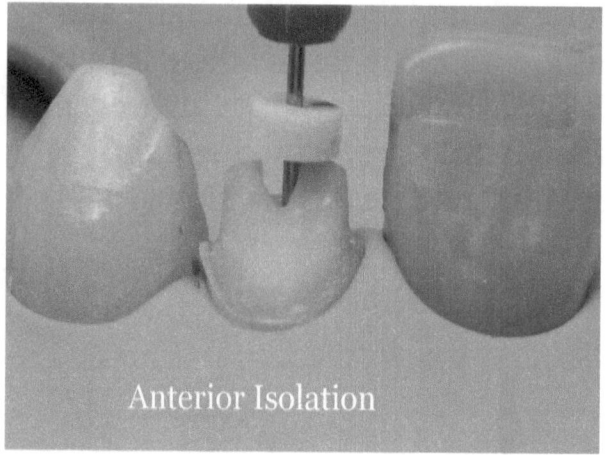

Anterior Isolation

Use
Green
stick
compound
to stabilize
the double
bowed
clamp
in Class V
isolation
the material
is placed over
and under the bow

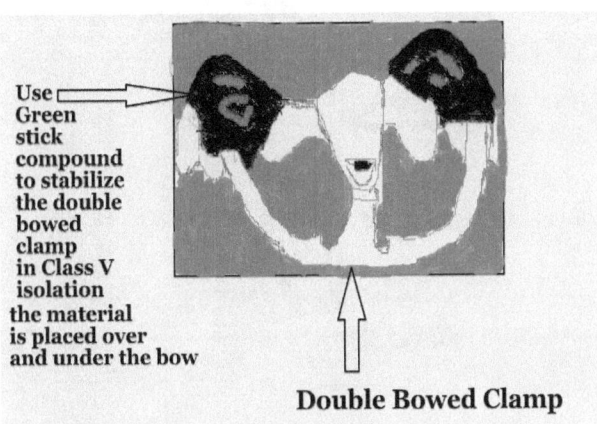

Double Bowed Clamp

Rubber Dam
Frame

Rubber Dam
sheet

Floss ligature

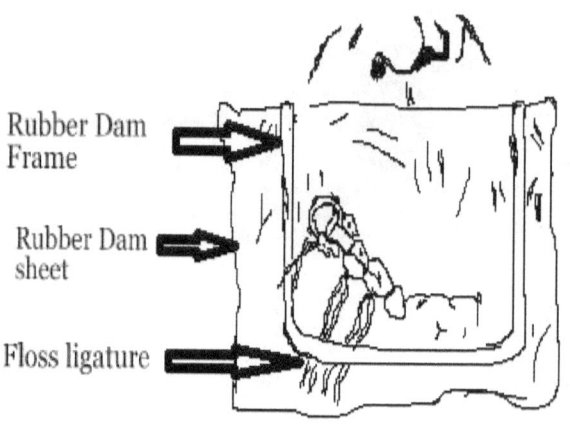

Rubber Dam in the Patient 's mouth

Acknowledgment

I would like to offer my deep, sincere
special thanks and appreciation to
Dr.Calogero Bugea who is an Italian oral
surgeon and endodontist for his
contribution with his photos and cases to
write this
glorious book .

References

Textbooks of Operative
Dentistry (with MCQ).

Textbook Of Operative
Dentistry 2nd edition ,Nisha
Garg and Amit Garg .

Summit's fundamentals Of
Operative Dentistry , 4th
edition .

Stuedvant Art and Science Of
Operative Dentistry ,sixth
edition .

Modern Operative Dentistry ,
Carlos Rocha .

Rubber Dam In Dentistry © 2020 Dr.Fawzia

Alht

www.ingramcontent.com/pod-product-compliance
Lightning Source LLC
Chambersburg PA
CBHW020603220526
45463CB00006B/2423